Your Healthy Child's Medical Workbook

Other books by Dylan Landis

Checklist for Your New Baby
Your Health and Medical Workbook
Your Healthy Pregnancy Workbook
Designing for Small Homes

Your Healthy Child's Medical Workbook

THE ESSENTIAL ORGANIZER FOR PARENTS

Dylan Landis

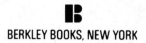

BERKLEY BOOKS, NEW YORK

This book is an original publication of The Berkley Publishing Group.

YOUR HEALTHY CHILD'S MEDICAL WORKBOOK

A Berkley Book / published by arrangement with
the author

PRINTING HISTORY
Berkley trade paperback edition / September 1997

The Putnam Berkley World Wide Web site address is
http://www.berkley.com

ISBN: 0-425-15982-5

BERKLEY®
Berkley Books are published by The Berkley Publishing Group,
200 Madison Avenue, New York, New York 10016, a member of Penguin Putnam Inc.
BERKLEY and the ''B'' design
are trademarks belonging to Berkley Publishing Corporation.

PRINTED IN THE UNITED STATES OF AMERICA

10 9 8 7 6 5 4 3 2 1

This health diary and medical workbook

contains the records of

_____

born _____

This book contains confidential and important
medical information. If found, please return to

_____

Address: _____

Phone: _____.

Contents

Acknowledgments

I am deeply indebted to two physicians: Jack T. Swanson, M.D., a member of the American Academy of Pediatrics Committee on Practice and Ambulatory Medicine, who patiently explained every test and vaccination; and Michael Traister, M.D., Assistant Professor of Clinical Pediatrics at the New York University School of Medicine, for his painstaking review of the manuscript and his many suggestions to improve it.

More information and ideas were kindly supplied by *Child* magazine and its former executive editor, Mary Beth Jordan; by Jerry Bowman, public relations manager for the American Academy of Pediatrics; and by Milcom, which makes medical record-keeping forms for doctors, and its parent company, Hollister.

Dominick Abel, my agent, has invested himself in all of my books, large and small, and I cannot thank him enough. Elizabeth Beier, my editor, has nurtured my three health workbooks from the beginning. Erica Landis had the excellent idea for the first workbook, which led to the series. Ari Baquet, my son, offered inspiration all around. Jan Gottlieb provided measureless support. I am grateful to them all.

How to Use This Book

When I gave birth to Ari seven years ago, my husband, Dean, and I knew nothing about babies. Thanks to the attentions of the nursing staff, we left the hospital with some basic information—like how to change a diaper, how to bathe a newborn, even how to start the paperwork for Ari's social security number.

But we never thought to ask his blood type or his Apgar score (a measure of his physical condition at birth), and we never kept any notes on his health care.

It was no surprise that I couldn't always give Ari's pediatrician fast, accurate information. I'd forget which antibiotic seemed to hurt his stomach. I'd forget the name of the prescription cough syrup that worked so well six months before. I honestly couldn't have told you the difference between one vaccination or another, and even whether Ari was up to date. (Fortunately, his pediatrician kept careful track.) And when Ari was sick, I often couldn't describe the course of his fever over more than a day or two, because I wasn't taking notes.

That's what it all boiled down to: keeping simple records. We weren't doing any of it. And since we moved three times before Ari was four years old, changing each time to a new pediatrician, we kept having to provide a new medical history from scratch. At times our memories, and our answers to a new doctor's questions, were pretty vague.

That's the whole point of writing things down.

What Makes This Workbook Different from Other Books on Children and Health?

Simply this: *You* write it.

When you visit or talk with the pediatrician, use this workbook to record your child's symptoms, your questions, the doctor's answers. Take notes on medications, so you can compare how they work (and any side effects).

If your child has a problem area—frequent stomachaches, perhaps, or signs of asthma—jot down your observations. If there's a pattern, you'll spot it fast, and that's information your doctor needs.

Your own records make this workbook valuable as a lifelong health document. Just fill in the blanks. Elaborate in the margins, if you like. The records start at birth, but you don't have to—begin at the appropriate point for your child.

And if a question or a chapter doesn't apply, pass it by.

Six Terrific Reasons to Keep Your Child's Medical Records

You'll remember information exactly when your doctor needs it. If you're stressed out or exhausted by a child's illness, how can you possibly recall all the details and facts? Having it all written down, along with a complete family medical history, is particularly valuable if you switch pediatricians or consult a new specialist.

You'll ask the right questions. Write questions down as they occur to you *before* visiting the pediatrician, so they won't be forgotten. Bring the book with you and note the answers. Now the information is permanently on file for your review. (Especially helpful if you take your child for a second opinion and want to compare what the doctors said.)

You might help your child stay healthier. Check the workbook for medically recommended schedules of checkups, tests and vaccinations. Even though your pediatrician is probably following the same schedule, your own records can help you keep your child's health care up to date.

You'll be more aware of good preventive medicine. By filling out the parents' medical history, you can spot patterns or conditions that might run in the family—and take action before a problem starts. At the very least, you'll be far more attuned to warning signs, which can mean earlier treatment—and faster recovery.

You'll have a record of medical bills and insurance payments. Now you can make sure you get every reimbursement and tax deduction you're owed.

You'll give your child a healthy start. This workbook will make up your child's own health record. With the records of treatments, medications, hospitalizations and the family history, it's a legacy of information your child can add to, and refer to, throughout his or her life.

Good health care is a gift we give our children. May this workbook help make your part easier.

Emergency Information and Fast Reference

Keep a photocopy of this worksheet where a baby-sitter, relative or doctor can easily find it: in a baby's diaper bag, a schoolchild's backpack, or luggage when appropriate.

Child's name _____ Date of birth _____

Address _____

Parents' telephone (day) _____ (home) _____

Person to contact in emergency _____

Medical conditions _____

Allergies (foods, medications, etc.) _____

Required daily medications and dosage _____

Other medications now being taken (use pencil) _____

Blood type _____

Hearing impaired? ☐ yes ☐ no

Use sign language? ☐ yes ☐ no

Medical insurance: Company _____

Telephone _____

Name of insured _____

Group no. _____ I.D. no. _____

Parent's Medical Release

If I cannot be reached in a medical emergency, I authorize *lifesaving* surgery to be performed on my child if medically necessary.

Signed _____

Print name _____

Relationship to child _____

Witness signature _____

Witness name (print) _____

The MedicAlert Bracelet

MedicAlert is a nonprofit, 24-hour service that can relay personal identification and medical facts over the phone to a hospital in case of emergency or accident. If your child has a medical condition or allergy, ask your pediatrician if a child-sized MedicAlert bracelet would be useful. (Enrollment is $35, plus a $15 annual fee; updates of your child's medical information are free and unlimited.)

For more information, call (800) 825-3785, or write

MedicAlert
2323 Colorado Avenue
Turlock, CA 95382

The simpler alternative: A few pharmacies sell bracelets that come pre-engraved with the name of a single allergy, such as penicillin; a jeweler can snip a few links to size it for your child's wrist. Or buy an ID bracelet from any jeweler and have it clearly inscribed. No 24-hour phone service backs up such a bracelet, but for a single allergy, it may be all your child needs.

Getting Organized

Address Book: My Child's Health Care Providers

Pediatrician _____

Telephone _____

Address _____

Other pediatricians in the practice or clinic _____

_____

Weekday hours _____

Weekend hours _____

Notes _____

_____

Backup pediatrician _____

(You may need a second pediatrician near grandparents' homes or a weekend house.)

Telephone _____

Address _____

Other pediatricians in the practice or clinic _____

_____

Weekday hours _____

Weekend hours _____

Notes _____

_____

Specialist (and specialty) _____

Telephone _____

Address _____

Referred by _____

Notes _____

_____

Specialist (and specialty) _____

Telephone _____

Address _____

Referred by _____

Notes _____

_____

Specialist (and specialty) _____

Telephone _____

Address _____

Referred by _____

Notes _____

_____

Pediatric dentist _____

Telephone _____

Address _____

Referred by _____

Notes _____

_____

Work and Insurance Contacts

Benefits advisor at Mom's workplace _____

Telephone _____

Address _____

Notes _____

Benefits advisor at Dad's workplace _____

Telephone _____

Address _____

Notes _____

Mom's insurance company or HMO _____

Group no. _____ I.D. no. _____

Telephone _____

Address _____

Notes _____

_____

Dad's insurance company or HMO _____

Group no. _____ I.D. no. _____

Telephone _____

Address _____

Notes _____

_____

Pharmacies

Consider opening a charge account at one or two pharmacies, including one that delivers. It may speed things up when you're home with a sick child.

Our local pharmacy _____

Address _____

Telephone _____

Hours _____

Notes _____

24-hour pharmacy _____

Address _____

Telephone _____

Notes _____

Pharmacy that delivers _____

Address _____

Telephone _____

Hours _____

Notes _____

Baby-sitters and Sick Child Care

Who can you call for relief if your child is sick? A few enlightened employers pay for visits by nurse's aides. It also helps to have a list of sitters whom you trust with medications, instructions and a feverish child.

Visiting nurse's aide service _____

Telephone _____

Notes on hours, fees and other arrangements _____

_____

Sitter _____ Telephone _____

Recommended by _____

What sitter charges _____

Notes _____

Sitter _____ Telephone _____

Recommended by _____

What sitter charges _____

Notes _____

Sitter _____ Telephone _____

Recommended by _____

What sitter charges _____

Notes _____

Sitter _____ Telephone _____

Recommended by _____

What sitter charges _____

Notes _____

Sitter _____ Telephone _____

Recommended by _____

What sitter charges _____

Notes _____

Sitter _____ Telephone _____

Recommended by _____

What sitter charges _____

Notes _____

Sitter _____ Telephone _____

Recommended by _____

What sitter charges _____

Notes _____

My Child's Former Pediatricians and Specialists

List any doctors who may have your child's old medical records on file. This information can be valuable to your current doctor, or to a new doctor if you move.

Pediatrician _____

Address _____

Telephone _____

Notes _____

Specialist _____

Address _____

Telephone _____

Notes _____

Specialist _____

Address _____

Telephone _____

Notes _____

Hotlines, Emergency Numbers and Other Resources

Pediatrician _____

Father's or partner's work number _____

Friends, neighbors, relatives I can call in an emergency

Name _____ home phone _____ work _____

Name _____ home phone _____ work _____

Name _____ home phone _____ work _____

Name _____ home phone _____ work _____

Ambulance _____

Police _____

Fire _____

Poison Control _____

(A state hotline, this number should be listed in the front of your local telephone directory; or call (800) POISON for the center nearest you. Post its number on your refrigerator.)

Other emergency numbers

Name: _____ Phone: _____

Name: _____ Phone: _____

Name: _____ Phone: _____

Name: _____ Phone: _____

Name: _____ Phone: _____

Name: _____ Phone: _____

Name: _____ Phone: _____

Name: _____ Phone: _____

Name: _____ Phone: _____

Name: _____ Phone: _____

Name: _____ Phone: _____

Name: _____ Phone: _____

Other hotlines

Name: _____ Phone: _____

Name: _____ Phone: _____

Name: _____ Phone: _____

Name: _____ Phone: _____

Name: _____ Phone: _____

Name: _____ Phone: _____

Name: _____ Phone: _____

Name: _____ Phone: _____

Name: _____ Phone: _____

Name: _____ Phone: _____

Name: _____ Phone: _____

Name: _____ Phone: _____

Information and Help by Phone

This is a slender sampling of the many groups that offer support and information. Your pediatrician may know of others, or you can look up organizations by subject in the *Encyclopedia of Associations* at any public library.

La Leche League (for breastfeeding support and information)
    National: (708) 455-7730
    Toll-free (but hard to get through): (800) LA LECHE

    Local contact _____
    and phone no. _____
(will be supplied by the national office)

ChildHelp USA (a 24-hour anonymous crisis and abuse hotline for overstressed parents)
    (800) 4-A-CHILD
    (800-422-4453)

Single Mothers by Choice (call for an information package)
    (212) 988-0993

National Organization of Mothers of Twins Club (call for a brochure and referral to local support group)
    (505) 275-0955

Parent Care (help for parents of premature and critically ill babies)
    (317) 872-9913

Depression After Delivery Support Network (volunteer-staffed; you may get a recording; call for literature, local support groups, the names of local therapists, etc.)
    (215) 295-3994

Perfectly Safe (a catalog of childproofing products)
    (800) 837-5437

Information to Write For

Allergy and asthma information—ask for a listing of publications and products, and a sample copy of this nonprofit organization's newsletter.

> Allergy and Asthma Network/Mothers of
> Asthmatics
> 3554 Chain Bridge Road, Suite 200
> Fairfax, VA 22030
> (800) 878-4403

Car seat information—a nonprofit group's guidance on how to choose and use car seats correctly. Write or call

> SafetyBeltSafe USA
> 123 West Manchester Blvd.
> Inglewood, CA 90301
> (310) 673-2666

Safe and Sound for Baby—a listing of products and home safety advice. Send self-addressed, stamped envelope to

> Juvenile Products Manufacturers Association
> P.O. Box 955
> Marlton, NJ 08053

Tips for Your Baby's Safety; The Safe Nursery; The Super Sitter—free brochures.

> The U.S. Consumer Products Safety Commission
> Publication Requests
> Washington, DC 20207

Is Your Crib Safe?—a brochure on crib safety, a potentially critical issue if you're borrowing a used crib. Free, but donations for this small, non-profit group are appreciated.

> The Danny Foundation
> 3158 Danville Blvd.
> P.O. Box 680
> Alamo, CA 94507
> or call (800) 83-DANNY

Manufacturers of Baby Goods and Gear

If you have questions about safety, sizes, warranties, nutrition or any other product information, you can get answers straight from the manufacturers just by picking up the phone. When you buy or borrow secondhand baby gear, call the manufacturer for a copy of the instructions.

A few companies, like Beech-Nut and Gerber, send out coupons and brochures on request. It can't hurt to ask.

Beech-Nut (800) 523-6633. Ask for the free "new parent pack."
Century (800) 837-4044, for product information and parts.
Cosco (800) 544-1108
Evenflo (800) 356-2229, for information on feeding supplies; (800) 233-5921, for furnishings.
Fisher-Price (800) 432-5437
Gerber Formula (800) 828-9119
Gerber Products Answer Line (800) 443-7237
Gerry (800) 525-2472
Graco (800) 345-4109
Playskool (800) 752-9755

Our Health and Life Insurance

Health Insurance or HMO Data

In an emergency or for hospital admissions, you may need this information fast.

Primary insurance company _____

Name of insured _____

Insured's social security no. _____

Child's social security no. _____

Group no. _____ I.D. no. _____

For doctor visits:

    Deductible _____ Co-payment _____

For hospitalization:

    Deductible _____ Co-payment _____

Our out-of-pocket maximum _____

Phone number to call for hospitalization approval _____

    Must phone within _____ hours for authorization

Phone number for general information _____

Where our insurance forms and data are filed _____

Secondary insurance company, if any _____

Name of insured _____

Insured's social security no. _____

Group no. _____ I.D. no. _____

For doctor visits:

    Deductible _____ Co-payment _____

For hospitalization:

    Deductible _____ Co-payment _____

Our out-of-pocket maximum _____

Phone number to call for hospitalization approval _____

    Must phone within ____ hours for authorization

Phone number for general information _____

Our HMO Information

HMO name _____

Member services telephone no. _____

Member I.D. (or social security) no. _____

HMO pediatrician _____

Address _____

Phone _____

Hospital affiliation _____

Notes _____

Child's HMO specialist, if any _____

Address _____

Phone _____

Notes _____

HMO pharmacy _____

Address _____

Phone _____

Hours _____ Do they deliver? ☐ yes ☐ no

Phone number to call for emergency medical

   treatment _____

   Call within ___ hours for emergency doctor's appointment

   Call within ___ hours for emergency hospitalization

   Where my HMO forms and data are filed _____

Medical Bills and Payments

Use these worksheets to track bills, payments and reimbursements. You may be able to deduct your unreimbursed medical expenses on your taxes, or perhaps you can deposit tax-free earnings into a flexible spending account to cover any unreimbursed expenses.

For submissions to a secondary insurance company or health care spending account, simply use separate lines.

Date of visit or test	Name of pediatrician or other provider	Amount of bill	Date I sent bill to insurance company	Amount reimbursed

Date of visit or test	Name of pediatrician or other provider	Amount of bill	Date I sent bill to insurance company	Amount reimbursed

Date of visit or test	Name of pediatrician or other provider	Amount of bill	Date I sent bill to insurance company	Amount reimbursed

Medical Bills and Payments   27

Date of visit or test	Name of pediatrician or other provider	Amount of bill	Date I sent bill to insurance company	Amount reimbursed

Date of visit or test	Name of pediatrician or other provider	Amount of bill	Date I sent bill to insurance company	Amount reimbursed

Date of visit or test	Name of pediatrician or other provider	Amount of bill	Date I sent bill to insurance company	Amount reimbursed

Checklist for a Safe Home

One of the best childproofing tests you can do is to think like a child yourself. On hands and knees, explore the house. What's under the sink, or just within reach? A number of innocuous objects can cause harm to a curious child—some even to a five-year-old who appears to be safety-conscious.

This abbreviated list of hazards is adapted from *The Perfectly Safe Home,* by Jeanne Miller (William Gray Publishing, $9.95; available through the Perfectly Safe catalog, [800] 837-5437).

To use the checklist, mark off any problems as you find and eliminate them.

☐ Plastic bags (a suffocation hazard; discard)

☐ Balloons (a choking hazard; store out of reach)

☐ Electrical outlets (fit with outlet covers)

☐ All cleaning supplies and polishes (store out of reach, or fit kitchen and bathroom cabinet doors with latches)

☐ Medications (fit medicine cabinet with latch before child is able to climb)

☐ Nearly all cosmetics and toiletries (fit bathroom cabinets with latches; fit bathroom door with childproof doorknob cover)

☐ Dangling cords from drapes or blinds (wind up, and place out of reach)

☐ Diaper pails and their deodorant cakes (keep pail tightly closed; consider placing pail in locked closet or childproof cupboard)

☐ Buckets or bowls of water; toilets (a drowning hazard for small children; use toilet latches or door locks to keep water inaccessible)

☐ Scalding tap or bath water (set thermostat for hot-water heater no higher than 120 degrees). *Note:* Safe bathwater temperature is 96 to 100 degrees; if you don't trust your hand as a guide, use a bath thermometer.

☐ Stairs (falling hazard for children ages one to four; block stairs with safety gates)

☐ Toys or household objects with small, detachable parts (good test: if it fits inside a toilet paper tube, it's a choking hazard to children under three years of age; store out of reach or discard)

☐ Tables or countertops with sharp edges (fit with padded corners or edges designed for childproofing)

☐ Windows (open from the top; fit with safety bars; keep locked when possible)

The Well-Stocked Medicine Cabinet

Note: Never give any oral medication to a child less than three months old without a pediatrician's approval.

- ☐ Non-aspirin pain and fever reliever (for infants *or* for children—don't confuse these different concentrations)

- ☐ Bacitracin antibacterial ointment

- ☐ 0.5% hydrocortisone cream for eczema or skin irritations (do not use on face or genitals unless recommended by your pediatrician)

- ☐ Band-Aids or other adhesive strips

- ☐ Oral antihistamine for insect bites or allergies, such as Benadryl or, in the generic, diphenhydramine, if recommended by your pediatrician

- ☐ Calamine lotion or other anti-itch cream

- ☐ Pediatric cold medicine, if recommended by your pediatrician

- ☐ Pediatric cough medicine, if recommended by your pediatrician

- ☐ Diaper rash medication, if recommended by your pediatrician

- ☐ Nasal aspirator, for unclogging infants' noses

- ☐ Saline nose drops to use with aspirator (first lubricate, then aspirate)

- ☐ Sunscreen, only for children older than six months, PABA-free and 15 SPF or higher

- ☐ Thermometer: Use a mercury rectal glass thermometer with children less than three months old, when accuracy is critical; digital thermometer is acceptable for older children (it beeps when ready, and is easier to read)

- ☐ Teething relief medication, if approved by your pediatrician

- ☐ Gauze pads

- ☐ Adhesive tape

☐ Tweezers

☐ First aid book or reference chart

☐ Ice pack (preferably instant-activating)

☐ Syrup of ipecac, to induce vomiting after certain types of poisoning. (*Note:* Never administer without instructions from your
local poison control center, as some poisons do twice the dam-
age if forced back up from the stomach.)

☐ Telephone number of poison control center (usually in front
pages of local telephone directory; post inside medicine cabinet, or on refrigerator door)

Background:
Family
Histories and
Childbirth Data

Mother's Medical History

This checklist can help reveal any medical conditions that run in the family, and that bear watching or preventive treatment in your child.

During pregnancy, did you:

Smoke? ☐yes ☐no How much? _____

Drink alcohol? ☐yes ☐no How much? _____

Take medications? If so, name them: _____

_____

Check under "Self" if you've ever had any of these conditions. For relatives, note the name and family relationship (sister, first cousin) under "Family." If you know the details of their conditions, treatment and outcome, write it down at the end of the section.

CONDITION	SELF	FAMILY
Alcoholism	☐	_____
Allergies or drug sensitivities	☐	_____
Anesthesia reactions	☐	_____
Anemia or blood disorders	☐	_____
Arthritis or joint problems	☐	_____
Asthma	☐	_____
Back problems	☐	_____
Birth defects or inherited diseases	☐	_____
Blood transfusions	☐	_____
Breast lumps or other problems	☐	_____
Breathing disorders (emphysema, bronchitis, etc.)	☐	_____
Cancer or tumors	☐	_____
Cough, persistant	☐	_____
Cystic fibrosis	☐	_____
Diabetes	☐	_____
Drug abuse	☐	_____
Depression	☐	_____
Eating disorders	☐	_____
Epilepsy or seizures	☐	_____
Exposure to chemicals or toxic substances	☐	_____
Exposure to DES during mother's pregnancy	☐	_____
Eye problems: retinitis pigmentosa	☐	_____
Gynecological conditions	☐	_____
Headache or migraine	☐	_____
Hearing problems: sensorineural deafness	☐	_____

CONDITION	SELF	FAMILY
Heart conditions	☐	_____
Hemophilia or clotting disorders	☐	_____
Hepatitis, jaundice or other liver disease	☐	_____
High blood pressure	☐	_____
Kidney or bladder problems	☐	_____
Mental retardation	☐	_____
Multiple gestation (twins, triplets)	☐	_____
Mumps, measles or chicken pox	☐	_____
Obesity	☐	_____
Pap smear irregularities	☐	_____
Psychological conditions	☐	_____
Phlebitis	☐	_____
Rheumatic fever	☐	_____
Rubella (German measles)	☐	_____
Skin problems, psoriasis	☐	_____
Sleep problems	☐	_____
Stomach, bowel or gallbladder problems	☐	_____
Stress, tension or anxiety	☐	_____
Stroke	☐	_____
Suicide or suicide attempt	☐	_____
Thyroid disease	☐	_____
Ulcer	☐	_____
Sexually transmitted diseases	☐	_____
Other _____	☐	_____
Other _____	☐	_____
Other _____	☐	_____

Causes of death: Mother's family

Record the cause of death, and age at death, for close relatives (grandparents, parents, siblings, children, aunts and uncles).

Maternal grandmother _____ age _____

Maternal grandfather _____ age _____

Paternal grandmother _____ age _____

Paternal grandfather _____ age _____

Mother _____ age _____

Father _____ age _____

Other close relatives _____ age _____

_____ age _____

_____ age _____

_____ age _____

Details and explanations

_____

_____

_____

_____

_____

_____

_____

_____

_____

_____

_____

_____

_____

_____

_____

_____

_____

_____

_____

_____

_____

_____

_____

Father's Medical History

This checklist can help you determine if any medical patterns run on Dad's side of the family. It could reveal conditions that run in the family, and that bear watching or preventive treatment in your child.

Check under "Self" if you've ever had any of these conditions. For relatives, note the name and family relationship (sister, first cousin) under "Family." If you know the details of their conditions, treatment and outcome, write it down at the end of the section.

CONDITION	SELF	FAMILY
Alcoholism	☐	_____
Allergies or drug sensitivities	☐	_____
Anesthesia reactions	☐	_____
Anemia or blood disorders	☐	_____
Arthritis or joint problems	☐	_____
Asthma	☐	_____

CONDITION	SELF	FAMILY
Back problems	☐	_____
Birth defects or inherited diseases	☐	_____
Blood transfusions	☐	_____
Breast lumps or other problems		_____
Breathing disorders (emphysema, bronchitis, etc.)	☐	_____
Cancer or tumors	☐	_____
Cough, persistant	☐	_____
Cystic fibrosis	☐	_____
Diabetes	☐	_____
Drug abuse	☐	_____
Depression	☐	_____
Eating disorders	☐	_____
Epilepsy or seizures	☐	_____
Exposure to chemicals or toxic substances	☐	_____
Exposure to DES during mother's pregnancy	☐	_____
Eye problems: retinitis pigmentosa	☐	_____
Gynecological conditions		_____
Headache or migraine	☐	_____
Hearing problems: sensorineural deafness	☐	_____
Heart conditions	☐	_____
Hemophilia or clotting disorders	☐	_____
Hepatitis, jaundice or other liver disease	☐	_____
High blood pressure	☐	_____
Kidney or bladder problems	☐	_____
Mental retardation	☐	_____

CONDITION	SELF	FAMILY
Multiple gestation (twins, triplets)		_____
Mumps, measles or chickenpox	☐	_____
Obesity	☐	_____
Psychological conditions	☐	_____
Phlebitis	☐	_____
Rheumatic fever	☐	_____
Rubella (German measles)	☐	_____
Skin problems, psoriasis	☐	_____
Sleep problems	☐	_____
Stomach, bowel or gallbladder problems	☐	_____
Stress, tension or anxiety	☐	_____
Stroke	☐	_____
Suicide or suicide attempt	☐	_____
Thyroid disease	☐	_____
Ulcer	☐	_____
Sexually transmitted diseases	☐	_____
Other _____	☐	_____
Other _____	☐	_____
Other _____	☐	_____

Causes of death: Father's family

Record the cause of death, and age at death, for close relatives (grandparents, parents, siblings, children, aunts and uncles).

Maternal grandmother _____ age _____

Maternal grandfather _____ age _____

Paternal grandmother _____ age _____

Paternal grandfather _____ age _____

Mother _____ age _____

Father _____ age _____

Other close relatives _____ age _____

_____ age _____

_____ age _____

_____ age _____

_____ age _____

Details and explanations

A Child's Earliest Medical History

Our baby's name _____

Where our baby was born: _____

   Hospital _____

   Address _____

Pregnancy Record

Note any tests that revealed problems during pregnancy, and use the section that follows for notes. (You don't need specific results of tests that went well.)

TEST	RESULTS
HIV	_____
Alpha fetoprotein	_____
Amniocentesis	_____
Chlamydia	_____

Chorionic Villus
  Sampling   _____

Fetoscopy   _____

Glucose tolerance _____

Gonorrhea   _____

Hepatitis B   _____

Herpes   _____

Iron level   _____

Non-stress test   _____

Sickle cell   _____

Syphilis   _____

Tay-Sachs   _____

Tuberculosis   _____

Sonogram   _____

Sonogram   _____

Sonogram   _____

OTHER TESTS   RESULTS

_____   _____

_____   _____

_____   _____

_____   _____

Notes and details on any problematic test results _____

_____

_____

_____

Childbirth Diary

Date of birth _____

Time of birth _____

Weight at birth _____

Length at birth _____

Hair color _____

Eye color _____

Birthmarks _____

Head circumference _____

Blood type _____

Pediatrician seen in hospital

　　Name _____

　　Address _____

　　Phone _____

Length of labor _____

Problems during labor _____

_____

☐ Vacuum used? ☐ Or forceps?

Details _____

_____

Medications used during labor _____

_____

Type of birth: ☐ vaginal ☐ c-section

Apgar score _____

The Apgar score is a rating of your baby's condition at birth; the highest score is 10. Up to two points each are given for baby's color, muscle tone, heart rate, respiratory rate and response to stimulus. Your baby actually gets two Apgar scores: the first at one minute after birth, the second at five minutes. Doctors combine the two scores into one with a slash. 8/9, for example, means the score rose from a healthy 8 to a very healthy 9.

Hereditary/metabolic screening or PKU test results:

☐ normal   ☐ abnormal
(Mothers who leave the hospital within twenty-four hours of childbirth will have to return, or see a pediatrician, to have this test taken.)

If abnormal, describe details and follow-up. _____

_____

Did baby experience any difficulties after birth?

☐ oxygen needed ☐ extra observation in special care nursery

Details _____

_____

How is my baby being fed?

☐ breast ☐ breast with supplementary bottles

☐ bottle   name and type of formula _____

If you're currently breastfeeding, describe the experience, including

both pleasures and problems. _____

_____

_____

_____

_____

Notes on the newborn physical exam:

Was jaundice noted? ☐ yes ☐ no

If yes, was blood test given for jaundice? ☐ yes ☐ no

   If yes, note peak bilirubin score. _____

Was hip click noted? ☐ yes ☐ no

Was heart murmur noted? ☐ yes ☐ no

Other comments _____

_____

_____

_____

_____

Notes:

How is your newborn sleeping and nursing in the hospital? How does he or she feel in your arms? Use this section for personal notes and reflections shortly after childbirth.

_____

_____

_____

_____

_____

_____

_____

_____

_____

_____

_____

_____

_____

_____

_____

_____

_____

_____

If Your Baby Was Adopted

Adoptive parents may have access to a good deal of medical information—or none at all. If you know one or both of your baby's biological parents, try to get them to fill out the Mother's Medical History (page 37) and Father's Medical History (page 42). If that's impossible, use this page to note any medical information you do have that may be useful to your baby later in life.

_____

_____

_____

_____

_____

_____

_____

_____

_____

_____

_____

_____

_____

_____

_____

_____

_____

_____

_____

_____

Baby Journal: Sleeping and Eating Habits

At certain stages of a child's life, sleeping and eating patterns—even if they're normal—can change, and cause some worry for parents.

The more hard information you can offer a doctor, the better he or she can reassure or advise you. For example, if your six-month-old cries endlessly at bedtime, take note of the situation *and* your own response; your pediatrician may spot a way to help break the pattern. If you worry (as some first-time mothers do) that your baby is not getting enough milk, note how long and how often the baby nurses, and discuss the results with your pediatrician.

Begin each section below with a date.

Date: _____   *Notes:* _____

_____

_____

_____

Date: _____ *Notes:* _____

_____

_____

_____

Date: _____ *Notes:* _____

_____

_____

_____

Date: _____ *Notes:* _____

_____

_____

_____

Date: _____ *Notes:* _____

_____

_____

_____

Date: _____ *Notes:* _____

_____

_____

_____

Date: _____ *Notes:* _____

_____

_____

_____

Date: _____ Notes: _____

_____

_____

_____

Date: _____ Notes: _____

_____

_____

_____

Date: _____ Notes: _____

_____

_____

_____

Date: _____ Notes: _____

_____

_____

_____

Date: _____ Notes: _____

_____

_____

_____

Date: _____ Notes: _____

_____

_____

_____

Date: _____ Notes: _____

_____

_____

_____

Date: _____ Notes: _____

_____

_____

_____

Date: _____ Notes: _____

_____

_____

_____

Date: _____ Notes: _____

_____

_____

_____

Date: _____ Notes: _____

_____

_____

_____

Date: _____ Notes: _____

_____

_____

_____

Date: _____   *Notes:* _____

_____

_____

_____

Date: _____   *Notes:* _____

_____

_____

_____

Date: _____   *Notes:* _____

_____

_____

_____

Date: _____   *Notes:* _____

_____

_____

_____

Date: _____   *Notes:* _____

_____

_____

_____

Date: _____   *Notes:* _____

_____

_____

_____

Hospitalizations and Special Conditions

Hospitalizations and Surgeries

The hospitalization of a child involves extraordinary stress for the family. Keeping records, even brief notations, will help you stay on top of the medical situation and give you a greater sense of control.

Your child's hospital records are filed under a patient record number. It's not essential, but if a doctor ever needs your file fast, having this number can speed up the process. You can get the number from your child's chart (just ask a nurse or intern), or by contacting the hospital later.

Use the separate Hospitalization Diary on page 63 to track any future hospital stay.

HISTORY OF HOSPITALIZATIONS

Date or year	Problem	Type of surgery or treatment	Doctor or surgeon	Hospital	Results and other notes	Patient record number

Notes _____

_____

_____

_____

_____

_____

_____

_____

_____

_____

_____

_____

_____

_____

A Hospitalization Diary

These worksheets cover tests, medications and day-by-day notes on a single hospital stay, should your child need one. Use the margins if you want to, and write down anything that seems important—it may be useful later.

If your child is in the hospital longer than six days, or more than once, photocopy the format for future use.

Tip: Mark this chapter with a bookmark or Post-it note, and leave it by your child's bedside. It could prove useful to a doctor if he or she needs answers and you're out of the room.

Reason for hospitalization _____

Hospital (address and phone) _____

_____

Date admitted _____ Date discharged _____

Patient record no. _____

Phone number of medical records dept. _____

Room no. _____ Room's phone number _____

Primary doctor _____

   Phone _____

Names of specialists, residents and other doctors seen in the hospital

_____   _____

_____   _____

Names of nurses and other staffers we want to remember

_____   _____

_____   _____

_____   _____

_____   _____

_____   _____

_____   _____

_____   _____

_____   _____

_____   _____

_____   _____

_____   _____

_____   _____

RECORD TESTS AND PROCEDURES

Date	Test or procedure	Who performed it	Why performed	Results	Side effects, if any

RECORD OF MEDICATIONS

Date	Medication	Dosage	Reason for Medication	Results	Side effects, if any

Journal Entries

Day 1

_____
Date

Doctor(s) seen today _____

What was discussed _____

What was decided _____

Overall, how did your child act, or seem to feel, today? _____

_____

Notes on fever, if any _____

Notes on diet _____

Notes on discomfort or pain _____

Questions to ask the doctor _____

_____

_____

_____

_____

_____

The doctor's answers _____

_____

_____

_____

_____

Day 2

_____
Date

Doctor(s) seen today _____

What was discussed _____

What was decided _____

Overall, how did your child act, or seem to feel, today? _____

_____

Notes on fever, if any _____

Notes on diet _____

Notes on discomfort or pain _____

Questions to ask the doctor _____

_____

_____

_____

_____

_____

The doctor's answers _____

_____

_____

_____

_____

Day 3

_____
Date

Doctor(s) seen today _____

What was discussed _____

What was decided _____

Overall, how did your child act, or seem to feel, today? _____
_____

Notes on fever, if any _____

Notes on diet _____

Notes on discomfort or pain _____

Questions to ask the doctor _____

_____

_____

_____

_____

_____

The doctor's answers _____

_____

_____

_____

_____

_____

Day 4

_____
Date

Doctor(s) seen today _____

What was discussed _____

What was decided _____

Overall, how did your child act, or seem to feel, today? _____

_____

Notes on fever, if any _____

Notes on diet _____

Notes on discomfort or pain _____

Questions to ask the doctor _____

_____

_____

_____

_____

_____

The doctor's answers _____

_____

_____

_____

_____

Day 5

_____
Date

Doctor(s) seen today _____

What was discussed _____

What was decided _____

Overall, how did your child act, or seem to feel, today? _____

_____

Notes on fever, if any _____

Notes on diet _____

Notes on discomfort or pain _____

Questions to ask the doctor _____

_____

_____

_____

_____

_____

The doctor's answers _____

_____

_____

_____

_____

_____

Day 6

_____
Date

Doctor(s) seen today _____

    What was discussed _____

    What was decided _____

Overall, how did your child act, or seem to feel, today? _____

_____

Notes on fever, if any _____

Notes on diet _____

Notes on discomfort or pain _____

Questions to ask the doctor _____

_____

_____

_____

_____

The doctor's answers _____

_____

_____

_____

_____

_____

Record of Special Medical Conditions

When you're following or treating a long-term condition such as asthma, allergies or headaches, you'll probably want extra space for notes. If a fever drags on for days, if your asthmatic child gets daily readings on a peak flow meter, or if you're trying to find a pattern in a series of headaches—this is the place to record your observations.

Structure your records as you wish. (You may want to borrow a format that's proved useful to you in another chapter.)

Tip: Start each entry with the date, and end it with any questions you want to remember to ask the pediatrician.

Date: _____ Notes: _____

_____

_____

_____

Date: _____ Notes: _____

_____

Date: _____ Notes: _____

_____

_____

_____

Date: _____ Notes: _____

_____

_____

_____

Date: _____ Notes: _____

_____

_____

_____

Date: _____ Notes: _____

_____

_____

_____

Date: _____ Notes: _____

_____

_____

_____

Date: _____ Notes: _____

_____

_____

_____

Date: _____ *Notes:* _____

_____

_____

_____

Date: _____ *Notes:* _____

_____

_____

_____

Date: _____ *Notes:* _____

_____

_____

_____

Date: _____ *Notes:* _____

_____

_____

_____

Date: _____ *Notes:* _____

_____

_____

_____

Date: _____ *Notes:* _____

_____

_____

_____

Date: _____   Notes: _____
_____
_____
_____

Date: _____   Notes: _____
_____
_____
_____

Date: _____   Notes: _____
_____
_____
_____

Date: _____   Notes: _____
_____
_____
_____

Date: _____   Notes: _____
_____
_____
_____

Date: _____   Notes: _____
_____
_____
_____

Date: _____ Notes: _____

_____

_____

_____

Date: _____ Notes: _____

_____

_____

_____

Date: _____ Notes: _____

_____

_____

_____

Date: _____ Notes: _____

_____

_____

_____

Date: _____ Notes: _____

_____

_____

_____

Date: _____ Notes: _____

_____

_____

_____

Date: _____ Notes: _____

_____

_____

_____

Date: _____ Notes: _____

_____

_____

_____

Date: _____ Notes: _____

_____

_____

_____

Date: _____ Notes: _____

_____

_____

_____

Date: _____ Notes: _____

_____

_____

_____

Date: _____ Notes: _____

_____

_____

Growth, Vaccinations, Tests and Medications: Medical Worksheets

MY CHILD'S GROWTH RECORD

Date	Age	Height	Weight	Head circumference	Blood pressure (after age three)

MY CHILD'S GROWTH RECORD

Date	Age	Height	Weight	Head circumference	Blood pressure (after age three)

Vaccinations and Tests

Vaccination Log and Worksheet

This schedule is recommended by the American Academy of Pediatrics. Ask your pediatrician to review it, however, before you fill it out, as the recommendations tend to change every couple of years. Your pediatrician may also want to vary the schedule slightly for your child.

Age	Vaccination	Date given
Birth to 2 months	Hepatitis B	_____
2 months	DTP, polio, Hib	_____
2 to 4 months	Hepatitis B	_____
4 months	DTP, polio, Hib	_____
6 months	DTP, Hib	_____
6 to 18 months	Hepatitis B, polio	_____

Age	Vaccination	Date given
12 months or older	VZV	_____
12 to 15 months	Hib, MMR	_____
12 to 18 months	DTP	_____
4 to 6 years	DTP, polio, possibly MMR	_____
11 to 12 years	MMR, if not given at 4 to 6 years	_____
11 to 16 years	Tetanus-diphtheria; hepatitis B if not given previously	_____

Note: Your pediatrician may also recommend a flu vaccine every year for a child with asthma or other medical conditions.

Key to the vaccinations

DTP: Diphtheria, Tetanus, Pertussis (whooping cough)
Hib: Hemophilus influenza type B (meningitis)
MMR: Measles, mumps, rubella
VZV: Varicella zoster virus (chicken pox)

ROUTINE SCREENING TESTS

Your pediatrician will schedule a number of the following tests. Some may be done repeatedly through childhood. Use this table to track results over time.

Key to the tests

Urinalysis: Tests for urinary infection and kidney abnormalities
Hematocrit or hemoglobin: Tests for anemia
Lead screening: Tests for lead poisoning
Metabolic screening: Tests for newborn heredity abnormalities, such as sickle cell anemia or PKU

Test	Date given	Results	Date given	Results	Date given	Results	Date given	Results
Urinalysis								
Hematocrit or hemoglobin								
Vision								
Hearing								
Lead screening								
Tuberculin test								
Cholesterol								
Dental checkup								
Other								
Other								

Date given	Results	Date given	Results	Date given	Results	Date Given	Results

Medication Log

Use this section to track the medications your child takes, including over-the-counter remedies. Feel free to track only those that concern you; for example, you may decide not to record cold and cough syrups, but take notes on antibiotics because of possible side effects or allergies.

The worksheet asks detailed questions, which can be helpful if your child takes several drugs at once, or periodically changes medications. Otherwise, just fill out the parts that seem most useful.

Remember to ask your doctor about any drug he or she prescribes: Are there side effects? Interactions with any other medications? Should the medication be taken with food? If you still have questions when you leave the office, ask your pharmacist, who should be able to give you complete information on any prescription drug.

RECORD OF MEDICATIONS TAKEN

Date	Medication	Why prescribed	Dosage & frequency	Side effects

RECORD OF MEDICATIONS TAKEN

Date	Medication	Why prescribed	Dosage & frequency	Side effects

RECORD OF MEDICATIONS TAKEN

Date	Medication	Why prescribed	Dosage & frequency	Side effects

RECORD OF MEDICATIONS TAKEN

Date	Medication	Why prescribed	Dosage & frequency	Side effects

Five-Year Journal of Doctor's Appointments

Checkup Schedule

You'll probably see a lot of the pediatrician, for everything from well-baby visits to a steady assortment of colds, ear infections and other minor illnesses.

The American Academy of Pediatrics suggests regular checkups for your child at the ages listed in the following table. (Your pediatrician may change the times to suit your child.) With only a couple of years skipped between ages six and ten, the checkups are annual.

Recommended age	Date of visit
Newborn (Usually performed in hospital)	_____
2 to 4 days (For babies discharged early from hospital)	_____
2 to 4 weeks	_____
2 months	_____
4 months	_____

Recommended age	Date of visit
6 months	_____
9 months	_____
12 months	_____
15 months	_____
18 months	_____
2 years	_____
3 years	_____
4 years	_____
5 years	_____
6 years	_____
8 years	_____
10 years	_____
11 years	_____
12 years	_____
13 years	_____
14 years	_____
15 years	_____
16 years	_____
17 years	_____
18 years	_____
19 years	_____
20 years	_____
21 years	_____

Diary of Pediatric Visits

Start each page *before* you see the pediatrician, noting your child's symptoms, if any, and questions you want to remember to ask. Bring this workbook to the doctor's office so you can take notes on the answers, or on treatment recommendations.

To extend the life of this workbook, you may want to leave one page of this diary blank and make photocopies as needed.

Reason for visit _____ **Date** _____

☐ checkup ☐ illness ☐ follow-up visit

Pediatrician seen _____

Describe problem, if any _____

Diagnosis _____

Treatment prescribed _____

_____

   (Note any medications prescribed on Medication Log, page 89.)

Tests performed, and results _____

_____

   (Note vaccinations on page 83–84, tests results on page 86–87.)

Questions to ask the pediatrician _____

_____

_____

_____

_____

Doctor's answers and advice _____

_____

_____

_____

_____

Recommended follow-up? _____

   (Note height, weight and other measurements in Child's Growth Record, page 81.)

Reason for visit _____ **Date** _____

☐ checkup ☐ illness ☐ follow-up visit

Pediatrician seen _____

Describe problem, if any _____

Diagnosis _____

Treatment prescribed _____

_____

   (Note any medications prescribed on Medication Log, page 89.)

Tests performed, and results _____

_____

   (Note vaccinations on page 83–84, tests results on page 86–87.)

Questions to ask the pediatrician _____

_____

_____

_____

_____

Doctor's answers and advice _____

_____

_____

_____

_____

Recommended follow-up? _____

   (Note height, weight and other measurements in Child's Growth Record, page 81.)

Reason for visit _____ **Date** _____

☐ checkup ☐ illness ☐ follow-up visit

Pediatrician seen _____

Describe problem, if any _____

Diagnosis _____

Treatment prescribed _____

_____

(Note any medications prescribed on Medication Log, page 89.)

Tests performed, and results _____

_____

(Note vaccinations on page 83–84, tests results on page 86–87.)

Questions to ask the pediatrician _____

_____

_____

_____

_____

Doctor's answers and advice _____

_____

_____

_____

_____

Recommended follow-up? _____

(Note height, weight and other measurements in Child's Growth Record, page 81.)

Reason for visit _____ **Date** _____

☐ checkup ☐ illness ☐ follow-up visit

Pediatrician seen _____

Describe problem, if any _____

Diagnosis _____

Treatment prescribed _____ ____

_____

(Note any medications prescribed on Medication Log, page 89.)

Tests performed, and results _____

_____

(Note vaccinations on page 83–84, tests results on page 86–87.)

Questions to ask the pediatrician _____

_____

_____

_____

_____

Doctor's answers and advice _____

_____

_____

_____

_____

Recommended follow-up? _____

(Note height, weight and other measurements in Child's Growth
Record, page 81.)

Reason for visit _____ **Date** _____

☐ checkup ☐ illness ☐ follow-up visit

Pediatrician seen _____

Describe problem, if any _____

Diagnosis _____

Treatment prescribed _____

_____

   (Note any medications prescribed on Medication Log, page 89.)

Tests performed, and results _____

_____

   (Note vaccinations on page 83–84, tests results on page 86–87.)

Questions to ask the pediatrician _____

_____

_____

_____

_____

Doctor's answers and advice _____

_____

_____

_____

_____

Recommended follow-up? _____

   (Note height, weight and other measurements in Child's Growth
Record, page 81.)

Reason for visit _____ **Date** _____

☐ checkup ☐ illness ☐ follow-up visit

Pediatrician seen _____

Describe problem, if any _____

Diagnosis _____

Treatment prescribed _____

_____

   (Note any medications prescribed on Medication Log, page 89.)

Tests performed, and results _____

_____

   (Note vaccinations on page 83–84, tests results on page 86–87.)

Questions to ask the pediatrician _____

_____

_____

_____

_____

Doctor's answers and advice _____

_____

_____

_____

_____

Recommended follow-up? _____

   (Note height, weight and other measurements in Child's Growth
Record, page 81.)

Reason for visit _____ **Date** _____

☐ checkup ☐ illness ☐ follow-up visit

Pediatrician seen _____

Describe problem, if any _____

Diagnosis _____

Treatment prescribed _____

_____

(Note any medications prescribed on Medication Log, page 89.)

Tests performed, and results _____

_____

(Note vaccinations on page 83–84, tests results on page 86–87.)

Questions to ask the pediatrician _____

_____

_____

_____

_____

Doctor's answers and advice _____

_____

_____

_____

_____

Recommended follow-up? _____

(Note height, weight and other measurements in Child's Growth Record, page 81.)

Reason for visit _____ **Date** _____

☐ checkup ☐ illness ☐ follow-up visit

Pediatrician seen _____

Describe problem, if any _____

Diagnosis _____

Treatment prescribed _____

_____

(Note any medications prescribed on Medication Log, page 89.)

Tests performed, and results _____

_____

(Note vaccinations on page 83–84, tests results on page 86–87.)

Questions to ask the pediatrician _____

_____

_____

_____

_____

Doctor's answers and advice _____

_____

_____

_____

_____

Recommended follow-up? _____

(Note height, weight and other measurements in Child's Growth Record, page 81.)

Reason for visit _____ **Date** _____

☐ checkup ☐ illness ☐ follow-up visit

Pediatrician seen _____

Describe problem, if any _____

Diagnosis _____

Treatment prescribed _____

_____

   (Note any medications prescribed on Medication Log, page 89.)

Tests performed, and results _____

_____

   (Note vaccinations on page 83–84, tests results on page 86–87.)

Questions to ask the pediatrician _____

_____

_____

_____

_____

Doctor's answers and advice _____

_____

_____

_____

_____

Recommended follow-up? _____

   (Note height, weight and other measurements in Child's Growth Record, page 81.)

Reason for visit _____ **Date** _____

☐ checkup ☐ illness ☐ follow-up visit

Pediatrician seen _____

Describe problem, if any _____

Diagnosis _____

Treatment prescribed _____

_____

   (Note any medications prescribed on Medication Log, page 89.)

Tests performed, and results _____

_____

   (Note vaccinations on page 83–84, tests results on page 86–87.)

Questions to ask the pediatrician _____

_____

_____

_____

_____

Doctor's answers and advice _____

_____

_____

_____

_____

Recommended follow-up? _____

   (Note height, weight and other measurements in Child's Growth
Record, page 81.)

Reason for visit _____ **Date** _____

☐ checkup ☐ illness ☐ follow-up visit

Pediatrician seen _____

Describe problem, if any _____

Diagnosis _____

Treatment prescribed _____

_____

   (Note any medications prescribed on Medication Log, page 89.)

Tests performed, and results _____

_____

   (Note vaccinations on page 83–84, tests results on page 86–87.)

Questions to ask the pediatrician _____

_____

_____

_____

_____

Doctor's answers and advice _____

_____

_____

_____

_____

Recommended follow-up? _____

   (Note height, weight and other measurements in Child's Growth
Record, page 81.)

Reason for visit _____ **Date** _____

☐ checkup ☐ illness ☐ follow-up visit

Pediatrician seen _____

Describe problem, if any _____

Diagnosis _____

Treatment prescribed _____

_____

   (Note any medications prescribed on Medication Log, page 89.)

Tests performed, and results _____

_____

   (Note vaccinations on page 83–84, tests results on page 86–87.)

Questions to ask the pediatrician _____

_____

_____

_____

_____

Doctor's answers and advice _____

_____

_____

_____

_____

Recommended follow-up? _____

   (Note height, weight and other measurements in Child's Growth
Record, page 81.)

Reason for visit _____ **Date** _____

☐ checkup ☐ illness ☐ follow-up visit

Pediatrician seen _____

Describe problem, if any _____

Diagnosis _____

Treatment prescribed _____

_____

(Note any medications prescribed on Medication Log, page 89.)

Tests performed, and results _____

_____

(Note vaccinations on page 83–84, tests results on page 86–87.)

Questions to ask the pediatrician _____

_____

_____

_____

_____

Doctor's answers and advice _____

_____

_____

_____

_____

Recommended follow-up? _____

(Note height, weight and other measurements in Child's Growth Record, page 81.)

110   Diary of Pediatric Visits

Reason for visit _____ **Date** _____

☐ checkup ☐ illness ☐ follow-up visit

Pediatrician seen _____

Describe problem, if any _____

Diagnosis _____

Treatment prescribed _____

_____

(Note any medications prescribed on Medication Log, page 89.)

Tests performed, and results _____

_____

(Note vaccinations on page 83–84, tests results on page 86–87.)

Questions to ask the pediatrician _____

_____

_____

_____

_____

Doctor's answers and advice _____

_____

_____

_____

_____

Recommended follow-up? _____

(Note height, weight and other measurements in Child's Growth Record, page 81.)

Reason for visit _____ **Date** _____

☐ checkup ☐ illness ☐ follow-up visit

Pediatrician seen _____

Describe problem, if any _____

Diagnosis _____

Treatment prescribed _____

_____

 (Note any medications prescribed on Medication Log, page 89.)

Tests performed, and results _____

_____

 (Note vaccinations on page 83–84, tests results on page 86–87.)

Questions to ask the pediatrician _____

_____

_____

_____

_____

Doctor's answers and advice _____

_____

_____

_____

_____

Recommended follow-up? _____

 (Note height, weight and other measurements in Child's Growth Record, page 81.)

Reason for visit _____ **Date** _____

☐ checkup ☐ illness ☐ follow-up visit

Pediatrician seen _____

Describe problem, if any _____

Diagnosis _____

Treatment prescribed _____

_____

 (Note any medications prescribed on Medication Log, page 89.)

Tests performed, and results _____

_____

 (Note vaccinations on page 83–84, tests results on page 86–87.)

Questions to ask the pediatrician _____

_____

_____

_____

_____

Doctor's answers and advice _____

_____

_____

_____

_____

Recommended follow-up? _____

 (Note height, weight and other measurements in Child's Growth
Record, page 81.)

Reason for visit _____ **Date** _____

☐ checkup ☐ illness ☐ follow-up visit

Pediatrician seen _____

Describe problem, if any _____

Diagnosis _____

Treatment prescribed _____

_____

(Note any medications prescribed on Medication Log, page 89.)

Tests performed, and results _____

_____

(Note vaccinations on page 83–84, tests results on page 86–87.)

Questions to ask the pediatrician _____

_____

_____

_____

_____

Doctor's answers and advice _____

_____

_____

_____

_____

Recommended follow-up? _____

(Note height, weight and other measurements in Child's Growth Record, page 81.)

114   Diary of Pediatric Visits

Reason for visit _____ **Date** _____

☐ checkup ☐ illness ☐ follow-up visit

Pediatrician seen _____

Describe problem, if any _____

Diagnosis _____

Treatment prescribed _____

_____

   (Note any medications prescribed on Medication Log, page 89.)

Tests performed, and results _____

_____

   (Note vaccinations on page 83–84, tests results on page 86–87.)

Questions to ask the pediatrician _____

_____

_____

_____

_____

Doctor's answers and advice _____

_____

_____

_____

_____

Recommended follow-up? _____

   (Note height, weight and other measurements in Child's Growth Record, page 81.)

Reason for visit _____ **Date** _____

☐ checkup   ☐ illness   ☐ follow-up visit

Pediatrician seen _____

Describe problem, if any _____

Diagnosis _____

Treatment prescribed _____

_____

   (Note any medications prescribed on Medication Log, page 89.)

Tests performed, and results _____

_____

   (Note vaccinations on page 83–84, tests results on page 86–87.)

Questions to ask the pediatrician _____

_____

_____

_____

_____

Doctor's answers and advice _____

_____

_____

_____

_____

Recommended follow-up? _____

   (Note height, weight and other measurements in Child's Growth Record, page 81.)

Reason for visit _____ **Date** _____

☐ checkup ☐ illness ☐ follow-up visit

Pediatrician seen _____

Describe problem, if any _____

Diagnosis _____

Treatment prescribed _____

_____

   (Note any medications prescribed on Medication Log, page 89.)

Tests performed, and results _____

_____

   (Note vaccinations on page 83–84, tests results on page 86–87.)

Questions to ask the pediatrician _____

_____

_____

_____

_____

Doctor's answers and advice _____

_____

_____

_____

_____

Recommended follow-up? _____

   (Note height, weight and other measurements in Child's Growth Record, page 81.)

Reason for visit _____ **Date** _____

☐ checkup ☐ illness ☐ follow-up visit

Pediatrician seen _____

Describe problem, if any _____

Diagnosis _____

Treatment prescribed _____

_____

   (Note any medications prescribed on Medication Log, page 89.)

Tests performed, and results _____

_____

   (Note vaccinations on page 83–84, tests results on page 86–87.)

Questions to ask the pediatrician _____

_____

_____

_____

_____

Doctor's answers and advice _____

_____

_____

_____

_____

Recommended follow-up? _____

   (Note height, weight and other measurements in Child's Growth Record, page 81.)

Reason for visit _____ **Date** _____

☐ checkup ☐ illness ☐ follow-up visit

Pediatrician seen _____

Describe problem, if any _____

Diagnosis _____

Treatment prescribed _____

_____

(Note any medications prescribed on Medication Log, page 89.)

Tests performed, and results _____

_____

(Note vaccinations on page 83–84, tests results on page 86–87.)

Questions to ask the pediatrician _____

_____

_____

_____

_____

Doctor's answers and advice _____

_____

_____

_____

_____

Recommended follow-up? _____

(Note height, weight and other measurements in Child's Growth Record, page 81.)

Reason for visit _____ **Date** _____

☐ checkup ☐ illness ☐ follow-up visit

Pediatrician seen _____

Describe problem, if any _____

Diagnosis _____

Treatment prescribed _____

_____

   (Note any medications prescribed on Medication Log, page 89.)

Tests performed, and results _____

_____

   (Note vaccinations on page 83–84, tests results on page 86–87.)

Questions to ask the pediatrician _____

_____

_____

_____

_____

Doctor's answers and advice _____

_____

_____

_____

_____

Recommended follow-up? _____

   (Note height, weight and other measurements in Child's Growth Record, page 81.)

120   Diary of Pediatric Visits

Reason for visit _____ **Date** _____

☐ checkup ☐ illness ☐ follow-up visit

Pediatrician seen _____

Describe problem, if any _____

Diagnosis _____

Treatment prescribed _____

_____

  (Note any medications prescribed on Medication Log, page 89.)

Tests performed, and results _____

_____

  (Note vaccinations on page 83–84, tests results on page 86–87.)

Questions to ask the pediatrician _____

_____

_____

_____

_____

Doctor's answers and advice _____

_____

_____

_____

_____

Recommended follow-up? _____

  (Note height, weight and other measurements in Child's Growth
Record, page 81.)

Reason for visit _____ **Date** _____

☐ checkup ☐ illness ☐ follow-up visit

Pediatrician seen _____

Describe problem, if any _____

Diagnosis _____

Treatment prescribed _____

_____

(Note any medications prescribed on Medication Log, page 89.)

Tests performed, and results _____

_____

(Note vaccinations on page 83–84, tests results on page 86–87.)

Questions to ask the pediatrician _____

_____

_____

_____

_____

Doctor's answers and advice _____

_____

_____

_____

_____

Recommended follow-up? _____

(Note height, weight and other measurements in Child's Growth Record, page 81.)

Reason for visit _____ **Date** _____

☐ checkup ☐ illness ☐ follow-up visit

Pediatrician seen _____

Describe problem, if any _____

Diagnosis _____

Treatment prescribed _____

_____

   (Note any medications prescribed on Medication Log, page 89.)

Tests performed, and results _____

_____

   (Note vaccinations on page 83–84, tests results on page 86–87.)

Questions to ask the pediatrician _____

_____

_____

_____

_____

Doctor's answers and advice _____

_____

_____

_____

_____

Recommended follow-up? _____

   (Note height, weight and other measurements in Child's Growth Record, page 81.)

Reason for visit _____ **Date** _____

☐ checkup ☐ illness ☐ follow-up visit

Pediatrician seen _____

Describe problem, if any _____

Diagnosis _____

Treatment prescribed _____

_____

   (Note any medications prescribed on Medication Log, page 89.)

Tests performed, and results _____

_____

   (Note vaccinations on page 83–84, tests results on page 86–87.)

Questions to ask the pediatrician _____

_____

_____

_____

Doctor's answers and advice _____

_____

_____

_____

Recommended follow-up? _____

   (Note height, weight and other measurements in Child's Growth
Record, page 81.)

Reason for visit _____ **Date** _____

☐ checkup ☐ illness ☐ follow-up visit

Pediatrician seen _____

Describe problem, if any _____

Diagnosis _____

Treatment prescribed _____

_____

    (Note any medications prescribed on Medication Log, page 89.)

Tests performed, and results _____

_____

    (Note vaccinations on page 83–84, tests results on page 86–87.)

Questions to ask the pediatrician _____

_____

_____

_____

_____

Doctor's answers and advice _____

_____

_____

_____

_____

Recommended follow-up? _____

    (Note height, weight and other measurements in Child's Growth Record, page 81.)

Reason for visit _____ **Date** _____

◻ checkup ◻ illness ◻ follow-up visit

Pediatrician seen _____

Describe problem, if any _____

Diagnosis _____

Treatment prescribed _____

_____

   (Note any medications prescribed on Medication Log, page 89.)

Tests performed, and results _____

_____

   (Note vaccinations on page 83–84, tests results on page 86–87.)

Questions to ask the pediatrician _____

_____

_____

_____

_____

Doctor's answers and advice _____

_____

_____

_____

_____

Recommended follow-up? _____

   (Note height, weight and other measurements in Child's Growth
Record, page 81.)

Reason for visit _____ **Date** _____

☐ checkup ☐ illness ☐ follow-up visit

Pediatrician seen _____

Describe problem, if any _____

Diagnosis _____

Treatment prescribed _____

_____

   (Note any medications prescribed on Medication Log, page 89.)

Tests performed, and results _____

_____

   (Note vaccinations on page 83–84, tests results on page 86–87.)

Questions to ask the pediatrician _____

_____

_____

_____

_____

Doctor's answers and advice _____

_____

_____

_____

_____

Recommended follow-up? _____

   (Note height, weight and other measurements in Child's Growth Record, page 81.)

Reason for visit _____ **Date** _____

☐ checkup ☐ illness ☐ follow-up visit

Pediatrician seen _____

Describe problem, if any _____

Diagnosis _____

Treatment prescribed _____

_____

   (Note any medications prescribed on Medication Log, page 89.)

Tests performed, and results _____

_____

   (Note vaccinations on page 83–84, tests results on page 86–87.)

Questions to ask the pediatrician _____

_____

_____

_____

_____

Doctor's answers and advice _____

_____

_____

_____

_____

Recommended follow-up? _____

   (Note height, weight and other measurements in Child's Growth
Record, page 81.)

Reason for visit _____ **Date** _____

☐ checkup ☐ illness ☐ follow-up visit

Pediatrician seen _____

Describe problem, if any _____

Diagnosis _____ / _____

Treatment prescribed _____

_____

(Note any medications prescribed on Medication Log, page 89.)

Tests performed, and results _____

_____

(Note vaccinations on page 83–84, tests results on page 86–87.)

Questions to ask the pediatrician _____

_____

_____

_____

_____

Doctor's answers and advice _____

_____

_____

_____

_____

Recommended follow-up? _____

(Note height, weight and other measurements in Child's Growth Record, page 81.)

Reason for visit _____ **Date** _____

☐ checkup ☐ illness ☐ follow-up visit

Pediatrician seen _____

Describe problem, if any _____

Diagnosis _____

Treatment prescribed _____

_____

   (Note any medications prescribed on Medication Log, page 89.)

Tests performed, and results _____

_____

   (Note vaccinations on page 83–84, tests results on page 86–87.)

Questions to ask the pediatrician _____

_____

_____

_____

_____

Doctor's answers and advice _____

_____

_____

_____

_____

Recommended follow-up? _____

   (Note height, weight and other measurements in Child's Growth
Record, page 81.)

Reason for visit _____ **Date** _____

☐ checkup ☐ illness ☐ follow-up visit

Pediatrician seen _____

Describe problem, if any _____

Diagnosis _____

Treatment prescribed _____

_____

   (Note any medications prescribed on Medication Log, page 89.)

Tests performed, and results _____

_____

   (Note vaccinations on page 83–84, tests results on page 86–87.)

Questions to ask the pediatrician _____

_____

_____

_____

_____

Doctor's answers and advice _____

_____

_____

_____

_____

Recommended follow-up? _____

   (Note height, weight and other measurements in Child's Growth Record, page 81.)

Reason for visit _____ **Date** _____

☐ checkup ☐ illness ☐ follow-up visit

Pediatrician seen _____

Describe problem, if any _____

Diagnosis _____

Treatment prescribed _____

_____

(Note any medications prescribed on Medication Log, page 89.)

Tests performed, and results _____

_____

(Note vaccinations on page 83–84, tests results on page 86–87.)

Questions to ask the pediatrician _____

_____

_____

_____

_____

Doctor's answers and advice _____

_____

_____

_____

_____

Recommended follow-up? _____

(Note height, weight and other measurements in Child's Growth Record, page 81.)

132   Diary of Pediatric Visits

Reason for visit _____ **Date** _____

☐ checkup ☐ illness ☐ follow-up visit

Pediatrician seen _____

Describe problem, if any _____

Diagnosis _____

Treatment prescribed _____

_____

   (Note any medications prescribed on Medication Log, page 89.)

Tests performed, and results _____

_____

   (Note vaccinations on page 83–84, tests results on page 86–87.)

Questions to ask the pediatrician _____

_____

_____

_____

_____

Doctor's answers and advice _____

_____

_____

_____

_____

Recommended follow-up? _____

   (Note height, weight and other measurements in Child's Growth Record, page 81.)

Reason for visit _____ **Date** _____

☐ checkup ☐ illness ☐ follow-up visit

Pediatrician seen _____

Describe problem, if any _____

Diagnosis _____

Treatment prescribed _____

_____

 (Note any medications prescribed on Medication Log, page 89.)

Tests performed, and results _____

_____

 (Note vaccinations on page 83–84, tests results on page 86–87.)

Questions to ask the pediatrician _____

_____

_____

_____

_____

Doctor's answers and advice _____

_____

_____

_____

_____

Recommended follow-up? _____

 (Note height, weight and other measurements in Child's Growth Record, page 81.)

134   Diary of Pediatric Visits

Reason for visit _____ **Date** _____

☐ checkup ☐ illness ☐ follow-up visit

Pediatrician seen _____

Describe problem, if any _____

Diagnosis _____

Treatment prescribed _____

_____

   (Note any medications prescribed on Medication Log, page 89.)

Tests performed, and results _____

_____

   (Note vaccinations on page 83–84, tests results on page 86–87.)

Questions to ask the pediatrician _____

_____

_____

_____

_____

Doctor's answers and advice _____

_____

_____

_____

_____

Recommended follow-up? _____

   (Note height, weight and other measurements in Child's Growth Record, page 81.)

Reason for visit _____ **Date** _____

☐ checkup ☐ illness ☐ follow-up visit

Pediatrician seen _____

Describe problem, if any _____

Diagnosis _____

Treatment prescribed _____

_____

   (Note any medications prescribed on Medication Log, page 89.)

Tests performed, and results _____

_____

   (Note vaccinations on page 83–84, tests results on page 86–87.)

Questions to ask the pediatrician _____

_____

_____

_____

_____

Doctor's answers and advice _____

_____

_____

_____

_____

Recommended follow-up? _____

   (Note height, weight and other measurements in Child's Growth Record, page 81.)

Reason for visit _____ **Date** _____

☐ checkup ☐ illness ☐ follow-up visit

Pediatrician seen _____

Describe problem, if any _____

Diagnosis _____

Treatment prescribed _____

_____

   (Note any medications prescribed on Medication Log, page 89.)

Tests performed, and results _____

_____

   (Note vaccinations on page 83–84, tests results on page 86–87.)

Questions to ask the pediatrician _____

_____

_____

_____

_____

Doctor's answers and advice _____

_____

_____

_____

_____

Recommended follow-up? _____

   (Note height, weight and other measurements in Child's Growth
Record, page 81.)

Reason for visit _____ **Date** _____

☐ checkup ☐ illness ☐ follow-up visit

Pediatrician seen _____

Describe problem, if any _____

Diagnosis _____

Treatment prescribed _____

_____

  (Note any medications prescribed on Medication Log, page 89.)

Tests performed, and results _____

_____

  (Note vaccinations on page 83–84, tests results on page 86–87.)

Questions to ask the pediatrician _____

_____

_____

_____

_____

Doctor's answers and advice _____

_____

_____

_____

_____

Recommended follow-up? _____

  (Note height, weight and other measurements in Child's Growth
Record, page 81.)

138   Diary of Pediatric Visits

Reason for visit _____ **Date** _____

☐ checkup ☐ illness ☐ follow-up visit

Pediatrician seen _____

Describe problem, if any _____

Diagnosis _____

Treatment prescribed _____

_____

   (Note any medications prescribed on Medication Log, page 89.)

Tests performed, and results _____

_____

   (Note vaccinations on page 83–84, tests results on page 86–87.)

Questions to ask the pediatrician _____

_____

_____

_____

_____

Doctor's answers and advice _____

_____

_____

_____

_____

Recommended follow-up? _____

   (Note height, weight and other measurements in Child's Growth Record, page 81.)

Reason for visit _____ **Date** _____

☐ checkup ☐ illness ☐ follow-up visit

Pediatrician seen _____

Describe problem, if any _____

Diagnosis _____

Treatment prescribed _____

_____

   (Note any medications prescribed on Medication Log, page 89.)

Tests performed, and results _____

_____

   (Note vaccinations on page 83–84, tests results on page 86–87.)

Questions to ask the pediatrician _____

_____

_____

_____

_____

Doctor's answers and advice _____

_____

_____

_____

_____

Recommended follow-up? _____

   (Note height, weight and other measurements in Child's Growth
Record, page 81.)

Reason for visit _____ **Date** _____

☐ checkup ☐ illness ☐ follow-up visit

Pediatrician seen _____

Describe problem, if any _____

Diagnosis _____

Treatment prescribed _____

_____

   (Note any medications prescribed on Medication Log, page 89.)

Tests performed, and results _____

_____

   (Note vaccinations on page 83–84, tests results on page 86–87.)

Questions to ask the pediatrician _____

_____

_____

_____

_____

Doctor's answers and advice _____

_____

_____

_____

_____

Recommended follow-up? _____

   (Note height, weight and other measurements in Child's Growth
Record, page 81.)

Reason for visit _____ **Date** _____

☐ checkup ☐ illness ☐ follow-up visit

Pediatrician seen _____

Describe problem, if any _____

Diagnosis _____

Treatment prescribed _____

_____

(Note any medications prescribed on Medication Log, page 89.)

Tests performed, and results _____

_____

(Note vaccinations on page 83–84, tests results on page 86–87.)

Questions to ask the pediatrician _____

_____

_____

_____

_____

Doctor's answers and advice _____

_____

_____

_____

_____

Recommended follow-up? _____

(Note height, weight and other measurements in Child's Growth Record, page 81.)

Reason for visit _____ **Date** _____

☐ checkup ☐ illness ☐ follow-up visit

Pediatrician seen _____

Describe problem, if any _____

Diagnosis _____

Treatment prescribed _____

_____

   (Note any medications prescribed on Medication Log, page 89.)

Tests performed, and results _____

_____

   (Note vaccinations on page 83–84, tests results on page 86–87.)

Questions to ask the pediatrician _____

_____

_____

_____

_____

Doctor's answers and advice _____

_____

_____

_____

_____

Recommended follow-up? _____

   (Note height, weight and other measurements in Child's Growth
Record, page 81.)

Reason for visit _____ **Date** _____

☐ checkup ☐ illness ☐ follow-up visit

Pediatrician seen _____

Describe problem, if any _____

Diagnosis _____

Treatment prescribed _____

_____

(Note any medications prescribed on Medication Log, page 89.)

Tests performed, and results _____

_____

(Note vaccinations on page 83–84, tests results on page 86–87.)

Questions to ask the pediatrician _____

_____

_____

_____

_____

Doctor's answers and advice _____

_____

_____

_____

_____

Recommended follow-up? _____

(Note height, weight and other measurements in Child's Growth Record, page 81.)

144   Diary of Pediatric Visits

Reason for visit _____ **Date** _____

□ checkup □ illness □ follow-up visit

Pediatrician seen _____

Describe problem, if any _____

Diagnosis _____

Treatment prescribed _____

_____

    (Note any medications prescribed on Medication Log, page 89.)

Tests performed, and results _____

_____

    (Note vaccinations on page 83–84, tests results on page 86–87.)

Questions to ask the pediatrician _____

_____

_____

_____

_____

Doctor's answers and advice _____

_____

_____

_____

_____

Recommended follow-up? _____

    (Note height, weight and other measurements in Child's Growth
Record, page 81.)

Medical Records to Carry When Traveling with a Child

Don't travel with this workbook; it would be hard to reconstruct if lost. Here are three ways you can keep your child's emergency medical history with you at all times:

• Have an emergency medical worksheet copied onto microfilm the size of a credit card. One company that does this commercially, supplying its own worksheet and charging $15, is

> AD Medical
> 315 Thorn Hill Lane, Suite 313
> Middletown, OH 45042

Note: Hospital staff may have to read the microfilm fast, so; type or write neatly on the worksheet.

• Carry a passport-sized booklet designed to hold a child's emergency medical data. The Children's Health Journal can be ordered for $3.95, plus 75 cents shipping and handling, from

> Informative Amenities, Inc.
> P.O. Box 1280
> Santa Monica, CA 90406

• Carry the credit card–sized EMX card, which is coded with your child's (or your own) medical history and bears a toll-free number. A hospital emergency room "reads" the card electronically or phones in for fast information. The annual cost: $45 for the first family member; $30 for each additional one. For information, contact

EMX
520 Madison Avenue
New York, NY 10022
(800) CALL EMX

About the Author

Dylan Landis writes books and magazine articles on health, children and interior design. She is a contributing editor for *Metropolitan Home,* writes a nationally syndicated column on design, and has been published in *House Beautiful* and *The New York Times* Home section. She lives in New York City with her husband and their son, Ari.